Home Care, Long-Term Care, Memory Care Units, and Other Living Arrangements

Laura Town and Karen Hoffman

Omega Press
Zionsville, IN 46077
© 2020 Omega Press

ISBN: 978-1-943414-13-0

Production Credits:
Authors: Laura Town and Karen Hoffman
Publisher: Omega Press
Photos: All credited images used under license from Shutterstock.com

Social media connections:

Laura Town
Twitter: @laurawtown
LinkedIn: https://www.linkedin.com/in/lauratown

Karen Hoffman
LinkedIn: https://www.linkedin.com/in/karen-hoffman-91502b62/

Omega Press in the News

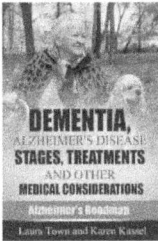

Dementia, Alzheimer's Disease Stages, Treatments, and Other Medical Considerations

- One of Book Authority's best books on dementia of all time
- One of Book Authority's best audiobooks on dementia of all time
- Audiobook recognized as a resource by the Alzheimer's Association
- Recommended by Dementia Insight
- Recommended by Alzheimer's Proof website
- Audiobook, ebook, and paperback available wherever books are sold

Long-Term Care Insurance, Power of Attorney, Wealth Management, and Other First Steps

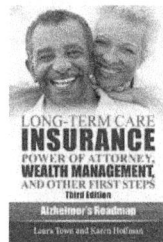

- One of Book Authority's best new insurance books to read in 2020
- Audiobook, ebook, and paperback available on Amazon

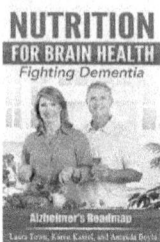

Nutrition for Brain Health: Fighting Dementia

- A Seniorlink (www.seniorlink.com) 50 Essential Read for Anyone Coping with Alzheimer's Disease
- Audiobook, ebook, and paperback available wherever books are sold

CONTENTS

Introduction

Alzheimer's disease is a progressive condition, worsening in terms of physical symptoms and cognitive decline as the disease moves into the later stages. If the disease is caught early enough, your loved one will likely continue daily activities without many changes to their routine or lifestyle. However, as the condition worsens, you will gradually need to make changes to ensure the safety and overall well-being of your loved one. These changes will at times be minor home repairs and precautions, but they could also include relocation and dedicated medical assistance. On average, individuals with Alzheimer's disease live 4 to 8 years past their diagnosis but may have as many as 20 years of remaining life. In these years, they will likely have to change living arrangements several times as the disease progresses. None of these changes are easy, and each one has its own unique challenges.

Living arrangements is a topic that should be discussed as early as possible so that your loved one can make their preferences known. In the early stages of the disease, your loved one can likely stay at home, but as the symptoms worsen, other options will need to be considered. For example, in my (Laura) situation, Dad lived at home independently for a short period of time, then he lived at home with us checking on him twice a day, then he had 24-hour at-home care, then he moved into an assisted living facility, and then he went into a nursing home. Each situation had its own financial and emotional stressors for me, my dad, and my family.

Currently, the nursing home population is 1.4 to 1.5 million people; in 2015, the number was 1.3 million. Not all of these people are elderly. According to statistics collected by the Centers for Medicare & Medicaid Services, 15.5% of this population are under the age of 65. The largest percentage (33.8%) of nursing home residents are age 85 to 94; the second-largest group (26.4%) are age 75 to 84. Given the broad age range the nursing home population represents, a person could be in a nursing home for 3 decades or more, depending on when they enter and how long they live.

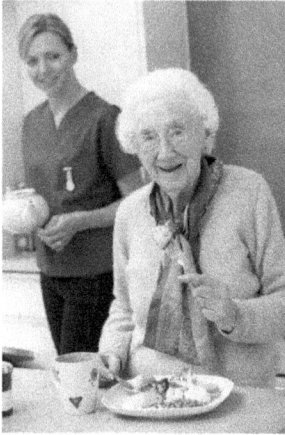
Credit: Monkey Business Images

Finding the living arrangement that works best for your loved one, as well as you and your family, is very important, and what is best will likely change as the disease progresses. Every situation is different, so while living with a caregiver might be the perfect option for one family, an assisted living facility or long-term care facility could be the best solution for another family. Before making these decisions, you should know the facts concerning each type of facility as well as some considerations involved in choosing the right facility. Alzheimer's disease has become much more prevalent in recent years. Therefore, many care providers and housing facilities have dedicated staff who are trained to work with individuals who have this disease. However, this is not always the case, so it is important to research the background and training of any facility you and your loved one are considering.

Chapter 1:
Staying at Home

Most of us would prefer to live in our homes unaided until our death. Although it is likely not possible for your loved one with Alzheimer's disease to do this, they will probably choose to stay at home as long they can. In the beginning, this will not involve a lot of planning or changes around the house, but as the disease progresses, changes will need to be made for both convenience and safety. Additional help may be needed around the house for daily cleaning tasks, laundry, maintenance, or companionship. When working with your loved one to make changes around the house or to their daily routine, try to ensure that these changes will not negatively impact their sense of independence. This can be difficult to balance, but preserving as much of their independence as possible will likely make a huge difference to your loved one.

Preserving Independence

Helping your loved one preserve their independence is important for someone in the early stages of Alzheimer's disease. This is important not only because your loved one will want as much independence as possible, but this also can help increase and preserve your loved one's mental acuity. You might feel compelled to take control of everything the moment your loved one is diagnosed with Alzheimer's disease because you think this will help relieve some of their burden or stress. In fact, the exact opposite is likely to happen. Upon being diagnosed with Alzheimer's disease, your loved one will begin to realize that soon it will be impossible to do many of the things they once enjoyed. This realization will turn any loss of independence, no matter how small, into a sign of what is to come in the future. The following checklist discusses tips for helping your loved one maintain independence while they still live at home.

Checklist: Helping preserve independence while living at home

- [ ] Stock the refrigerator and pantries with easy-to-make foods, such as sandwich materials or meals that can be made in the microwave. If your loved one has experienced problems using the microwave, consider posting directions for microwave use nearby (see *Home Safety Checklist Guide and Caregiver Resources for Medication Safety, Driving, and Wandering*).

- [ ] If your loved one enjoys cooking, offer to help them cook a few meals each week, but make sure not to take over. Allow your loved one to do as much of the preparation as possible, only lending support when necessary.

- [ ] If your loved one can no longer cook and you are not able to help, arrange with Meals on Wheels to deliver hot meals to your loved one.

- [ ] Help your loved one set up automatic bill payments for their monthly bills.

- [ ] For bills that cannot be set up through bill pay (snow removal, local newspaper delivery, landscaping, etc.), suggest that your loved one create a calendar with dates for when these payments need to be made. Once the check is delivered, your loved one can check it off on the calendar.

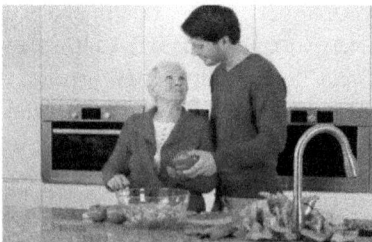

Credit: Photographee.eu

4

- ☐ Help your loved one set up daily routines to make the management of daily tasks easier and less stressful.

- ☐ If your loved one is used to doing the grocery shopping, help them create a grocery list so the trip is easier.

- ☐ If becoming confused at the grocery store is a concern, offer to go with your loved one. Be there for support and companionship, but do not interfere unless they need or ask for your help. Alternately, you could help your loved one create an online shopping list and have the groceries delivered to their home.

- ☐ Buy an electric tea kettle so that your loved one can make tea or instant coffee without having to worry about forgetting the stove is on. Make sure you purchase a device with an automatic shut-off feature.

- ☐ Be observant about tasks that are going undone in your loved one's home (e.g., cleaning, laundry, grocery shopping) and offer to help. Your loved one may be resistant to ask for help with everyday tasks, but if you offer, they may be less hesitant to accept.

- ☐ Post clear instructions for common appliances such as the washing machine and dryer, stove/oven, dishwasher, telephone, TV, shower or bath, and toilet. This will help your loved one know how to use these appliances if they get confused or can't remember.

- ☐ If your loved one has trouble with incontinence, place incontinence pads close to the toilet for your loved one to use.

☐ Avoid taking control. In the early stages of Alzheimer's disease, your loved one can still do many things on their own, so only offer help when needed.

☐ If your loved one used to enjoy going for walks (or other similar activities) but has stopped due to a fear of getting confused or lost, offer to go for a walk with them on a set day or two each week.

☐ If your loved one has a pet, post reminders to feed the pet, take it outside to use the bathroom, or other needed pet chores.

☐ For more information about helping your loved one maintain their independence, see *Caregiver Resources for Helping with Activities of Daily Living.*

Meals on Wheels

Meals on Wheels America is a senior nutrition program that works to ensure no elder adult goes without food. Approximately 1 million meals per day are provided by Meals on Wheels in the United States, with options to deliver either breakfast, lunch, or dinner. These meals are served at senior centers or can be delivered straight to a person's home. If your loved one has Alzheimer's disease and does not cook anymore (either for safety reasons or because they do not want to), signing them up for Meals on Wheels could be a good solution. The checklist below discusses some of the aspects of this program.

Checklist: Basics about the Meals on Wheels program

☐ The individual receiving meals must be homebound (not able to leave the home, or it is difficult to leave the home) and at least 60 years old.

☐ Those under 60 can also receive meals if they have a disability or their income is low enough to meet the requirements. These requirements often differ by state and program, so check with your local organization to see if your loved one qualifies.

- [ ] You can sign a loved one up to have meals delivered to their house; individuals do not have to sign themselves up for the program.

- [ ] Prices per meal vary by state but are often less than $8 a meal.

- [ ] Some areas offer meal packages where you can pay for meals by the week.

- [ ] You will need to fill out an application (or answer questions over the phone) regarding any dietary restrictions you loved one has.

- [ ] Meals on Wheels programs employ nutritionists, so meals are healthy and well balanced. All meals meet the dietary guidelines of the Older Americans Act Nutrition Program and are designed to adhere to the medical needs and cultural preferences of the individual.

- [ ] Some programs will also provide pet food at a discounted rate once a month for seniors who have pets living with them.

- [ ] In some areas, Meals on Wheels programs offer grocery shopping services to homebound seniors.

- [ ] For individuals who have meals delivered weekly, non-perishable food items are delivered in advance of very bad weather. This way, if a volunteer cannot make it to your loved one's home because of the weather, food is still available.

- [ ] Meals are generally only served on weekdays (Monday–Friday), but frozen meals can be provided for the weekends if needed.

- ☐ Once you sign your loved one up, meal delivery can generally start within a day or two. It may take longer in some areas, but they try to start as soon as possible.

- ☐ Meals on Wheels has programs across the country in both rural and urban areas. You can visit their website to find a provider near you. Additional contact information for this program can be found in the Resources at the end of the book.

Home Modifications

In order for your loved one to safely stay in their home, you may need to make several modifications. These changes are made not only for your loved one's safety but also to increase their independence and overall well-being. Changes to the house can be expensive, but they are necessary and can prevent greater expenses later on. Some changes that should be made for safety include locking up medications and hazardous products such as cleaning solutions and guns. Other safety-related modifications are made to prevent falling, tripping, and wandering. For a full list of safety changes, please see *Home Safety Checklist Guide and Caregiver Resources for Medication Safety, Driving, and Wandering*.

In addition to home safety modifications, changes can also be made to reduce disorientation and promote independence. The following checklist details some changes that can be made to the home.

Checklist: Home modifications to reduce confusion

- ☐ Have an accurate clock in every room so your loved one can be aware of the passing of time and use it to orient their mind to the time of day.

- ☐ Hang a calendar with large numbers in the room in which your loved one spends the most time. You or your loved one can cross days off as they pass, and you can also add appointments to the calendar to help your loved one remember them.

☐ Avoid rearranging rooms in the house unless the change is needed for safety reasons.

☐ Purchase a digital voice reminder device for the door your loved one uses to exit the house. These reminders will sound when the door opens; a voice recording will instruct your loved one to turn off the lights and remember the house keys, or whatever messages you program into the device.

☐ Hang signs with the room name on or next to the door for common rooms, such as the bedroom, bathroom, and kitchen. This will help your loved one find the needed room if they get disoriented. If needed, add an explanation of the purpose of the room.

☐ Close doors and post "keep out" signs for rooms that your loved one does not need to use.

☐ Get rid of excess or unneeded clothing to decrease choices, which will help eliminate some stress.

☐ Remove all excess clutter from the house.

☐ Ensure that stairways are well lit; this could include adding light switches at the top and bottom of each stairwell.

☐ Add reflective and/or colorful tape to the edge of stairs to increase visibility.

☐ Install extra lighting in all rooms.

Home Services

While your loved one is living at home, you may find it beneficial to look into home service options. During the early stages of the disease, your loved one will likely not need medical services or help with personal care unless there are other preexisting conditions, but they may benefit from companion services or homemaker services. Companion services can be arranged for once a week or

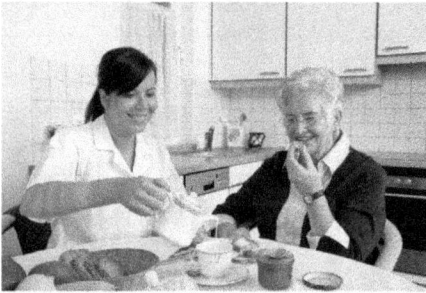
Credit: Lisa S.

multiple times a week, as needed. If your loved one is living with their spouse or another family member, then perhaps they only need someone to come in once or twice a week. Homemaker services provide help with cooking, cleaning, laundry, food shopping, and other similar tasks. Even if your loved one is independent enough to live at home, and possibly alone, both of these services can be helpful to decrease loneliness and frustration. If your loved one has always done the cooking and cleaning but is no longer able to perform these tasks all the time, they may become easily frustrated when they are unable to successfully complete these tasks alone. To find local home service providers in your area, consult the Resources at the end of the book. The checklist below discusses the duties performed by different home service providers.

Checklist: Types of duties performed by home services

Homemaker Services:

☐ Cooking

- ☐ Washing dishes
- ☐ Laundry
- ☐ Changing bed sheets
- ☐ Dusting
- ☐ Vacuuming
- ☐ Cleaning bathrooms
- ☐ Taking out trash
- ☐ Organization
- ☐ Medicine schedule reminders
- ☐ Pet care
- ☐ Houseplant care
- ☐ Errand assistance
- ☐ Grocery shopping

Companion Services:

- ☐ Conversation
- ☐ Recreational activities (games, movies, walks, favorite hobbies, puzzles, etc.)
- ☐ Transportation to doctor's appointments or the grocery store
- ☐ Assistance in running errands
- ☐ Cognitive stimulation
- ☐ Help with phone calls
- ☐ Help with email or letter writing
- ☐ Light cleaning and cooking

Personal Care Services:

- ☐ Assistance with bathing

- ☐ Assistance with dressing
- ☐ Assistance with toileting
- ☐ Feeding assistance and monitoring
- ☐ Medicine reminders and monitoring
- ☐ Cooking
- ☐ Cleaning
- ☐ Laundry
- ☐ Changing bed sheets
- ☐ Shopping
- ☐ Providing transportation to appointments or the grocery store

Every Alzheimer's patient is unique in their needs and daily struggles. Therefore, there are no specific guidelines as to when your loved one will need different types of home services. The following checklist describes some indicators that your loved one may be in need of additional help around the house.

Checklist: When should my loved one start receiving home services?

- ☐ The laundry is piling up without being washed.
- ☐ You notice that your loved one wears clothes repeatedly without laundering them.
- ☐ Your loved one has not changed the bed sheets in weeks.
- ☐ Your loved one has started sleeping on the couch because the bed sheet and/or blankets need to be washed.
- ☐ The sink is always full of dirty dishes.

- You notice that many dishes are broken or misplaced.

- The refrigerator has an abundance of old and/or spoiled food.

- The cupboards contain mostly old or expired food.

- There is very little food in the house because your loved one has not gone grocery shopping.

- Your loved one is going without eating because they do not want to cook.

- Your loved one has a pet whose food dish is empty most times when you visit.

- Your loved one has difficulty bathing and/or dressing and is resistant to asking you or another family member for help.

- You notice that your loved one has bruises or injuries from falling when getting into or out of the shower or bathtub.

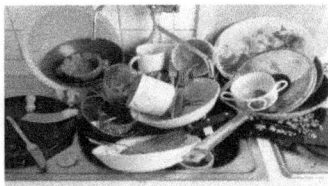

Credit: Camilo

- Extra medication is present in your loved one's pill organizer because they have forgotten to take their pills multiple times.

- Unopened letters and correspondence pile up around the house.

- Your loved one resists asking you for help with tasks around the house.

- Your loved one's house has fallen well below the level of cleanliness your loved one maintained before becoming ill.

- A layer of dust is present on tables, bookshelves, and other stationary items.

- Newspapers and other recyclables have started piling up.

- The carpet appears to not have been vacuumed in weeks, if not longer.

- The floors are covered with mud, dirt, and debris from a lack of sweeping and mopping.

- You realize that your loved one has very little social interaction and spends most days only watching television.

- The only person your loved one talks to most weeks is you.

- Your loved one frequently complains about feeling lonely.

- Your loved one is no longer able to drive but has various appointments during the day.

You do not need to arrange companion and homemaker services through an agency or outside source. A relative, family member, friend, or neighbor could stop by a few times a week to visit your loved one and help around the house. If you or your loved one has a large support network close by, such as friends, relatives, church companions, and/or community members, you can create a Caring Bridge website to set up a schedule of what everyone can do to help. (Please see the Resources for more information.) This approach could ultimately relieve a lot of your stress. However, a large support group is not always available, so you also have the option to hire someone to perform these tasks. Both independent employees and caregiver service organizations are available; you can also sometimes find help through local churches, colleges with social work and nursing majors, senior centers, and community aid agencies. Before hiring someone for these positions, you should go through a thorough interview process. Consider the following checklist of questions to ask during an interview.

Checklist: Questions to ask when hiring companion and homemaker services

- ☐ What is their previous work experience?
- ☐ Have they worked with someone with Alzheimer's disease before?
- ☐ Will they submit to a background check?
- ☐ Do they have references?
- ☐ Have they ever been fired from a home service position before? If so, what was the reason for termination?
- ☐ In order to ensure they get along well with your loved one, are they willing to be hired on a trial basis first?
- ☐ Would your loved one prefer someone of the same gender to provide care, especially if they will be helping with bathing or dressing?
- ☐ Do they seem responsible? Have they answered all phone calls and/or emails in a timely manner? Did they show up to the interview on time?
- ☐ Do they have an agreeable personality/attitude?
- ☐ Do they appear to be patient?
- ☐ If they are interviewing to be a companion, what activities do they plan to do?
- ☐ Can they adjust their cooking style to meet the dietary needs of your loved one?
- ☐ Are they CPR and/or first aid certified?

- [ ] If they are applying to a position in which they will be driving your loved one, how is their driving record?

- [ ] Do they have a reliable form of transportation? Do they have car insurance?

- [ ] If they are applying for a position where they will be expected to clean, are there any tasks they will not do? For example, are they opposed to cleaning toilets or washing dishes by hand?

Home Healthcare

Once your loved one progresses to the mid to late stages of Alzheimer's disease, they will likely need home healthcare services. Home healthcare could also be beneficial to your loved one in the earlier stages of the disease, especially if they have a preexisting condition or have difficulty taking medications properly. Home healthcare services are generally provided by a nurse or physician's assistant and can help with administering medications, bathing, eating, and sometimes even physical therapy. Home healthcare can be provided in your loved one's home as often as they need the services. The aide can visit weekly, daily, or even provide 24-hour-a-day care. If around-the-clock service is provided, this will generally allow your loved one to stay in their home longer, avoiding the need to move in with a caregiver.

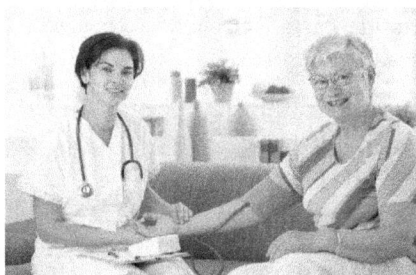

Credit: StockLite

Checklist: When to hire home healthcare

☐ Your loved one needs help with medications.

☐ Your loved one needs wound care.

☐ Your loved one is experiencing medical problems beyond your abilities, especially medical problems in addition to Alzheimer's disease (e.g., diabetes, heart disease, or blood clots).

☐ Your loved one needs daily or weekly injections.

☐ Your loved one gets infections easily.

☐ Your loved one requires specialized medical equipment.

☐ You are making frequent visits to the doctor for things that could be handled by a nurse at your home.

☐ Your loved one has particular diet and nutritional needs.

☐ Your loved one needs help bathing and dressing.

☐ Your loved one requires physical therapy.

Before hiring someone to work with your loved one, you should do some research into the company or service you are considering. Some Resources to help with this research are included at the end of the book. The following checklist discusses what to look for when hiring home healthcare.

Checklist: What to look for when hiring home healthcare

☐ Does the healthcare service run background checks on their employees?

☐ Are the employees trained to care for patients with Alzheimer's disease?

- [ ] What kind of training do the employees receive?
- [ ] What skill level are the employees? RNs? CNAs?
- [ ] How are the employees monitored to ensure a high quality of care?
- [ ] What policies are in place to handle problems if they arise?
- [ ] Will you be able to personally choose/interview the employees who will be working with your loved one?
- [ ] Will they take patients who are incontinent?
- [ ] Can the home healthcare worker take your loved one to the hospital if necessary, or will an ambulance need to be called?
- [ ] Will the home healthcare worker wait with your loved one until you get to the hospital?
- [ ] Will you need to provide meals for the home healthcare worker, or will they bring their own?
- [ ] Is it possible to do a trial day/week to see how the employee and your loved one interact together?
- [ ] Will your loved one be assigned a regular healthcare worker or will the person change each week/day?
- [ ] If a regular healthcare worker is not available to come due to illness or other factors, will a replacement be sent?
- [ ] How will you be notified of the replacement?
- [ ] How long has the company been in business?
- [ ] What kind of reputation do they have within the community?
- [ ] Is the service only available during the week, or do they have weekend care as well?

- ☐ Is the company an approved Medicare or Medicaid provider?

- ☐ Does the company honor the Patient's Bill of Rights (the patient's overall rights in terms of care, such as being treated with respect)?

- ☐ Will the company provide you with a sample plan of care for a client with Alzheimer's disease?

- ☐ What is the company's policy on patient confidentiality?

- ☐ Are fees fixed or do they work on a sliding scale?

- ☐ Is there financial assistance available when needed?

- ☐ Is the company licensed by the state?

- ☐ Do the company's representatives seem friendly and helpful?

- ☐ Does the company have relationships with dietitians, counselors, and/or other specialists? Can they provide referrals if/when they are needed?

- ☐ How quickly do services begin?

Geriatric Care Manager

When you feel it is time to hire home services, consider finding a geriatric care manager who will oversee your loved one's home care. Geriatric care managers are generally social workers, counselors, nurses, or other professionals in the field of geriatrics (a branch of medicine specializing in the care of older adults). The role of a geriatric care manager is to aid families and their loved ones with the many challenges associated with finding appropriate care. For your loved one with Alzheimer's disease, a care manager would get to know your loved one as well as the family and then work to suggest the best care in terms of insurance, resources, and the reputation of the facility, if applicable. These managers facilitate care, whether in the home or in a residential facility. If, as a caregiver, you are overwhelmed by determining the best living arrangements for your loved one, or you are unsure if your loved one's current living arrangements are in their best interest, you may want to consider a geriatric care manager.

Geriatric care managers are rarely, if ever, covered by insurance companies or Medicare, and their fees may prohibit you from considering this option. However, sometimes a sliding scale fee can be arranged depending on the company or individual being hired. If you are interested in this type of service, conduct research to find an agency that provides the services you want at the best price. The checklists below discuss the services that most geriatric care managers offer, signs to help you determine which services might be of use to you, and what to look for in a care manager.

Checklist: What services do geriatric care managers provide?

- [ ] Customize all services and suggestions specifically to your loved one's needs by performing in-depth interviews with caregivers, family, and your loved one.

- [ ] Recommend a care plan tailored to your loved one's needs.

- [ ] Set up and attend doctor's appointments with your loved one.

- [ ] Ensure communication between doctors and your loved one and family.

- [ ] Act as an advocate for you and your loved one in cases where there are disagreements with a living facility, hospital, or doctor.

- [ ] Manage your loved one's medication schedule.

- ☐ Help plan for the future needs of your loved one based on the progression of the disease.

- ☐ Help avoid preventable or unnecessary hospitalization, incorrect placements, and/or duplicated services.

- ☐ Suggest the most appropriate forms of home care services needed.

- ☐ Suggest measures that can be taken to make your loved one's environment safer as the disease progresses.

- ☐ Recommend and facilitate social and recreational activities.

- ☐ Monitor your loved one's condition and suggests changes in housing arrangements and/or services when necessary.

- ☐ Help select living arrangements and organize all details to facilitate the move.

- ☐ Help smooth transitions between living situations.

- ☐ Provide crisis intervention and counseling, as needed.

- ☐ Recommend legal assistance by working with elder care attorneys (see *Advance Directives, Durable Power of Attorney, Wills, and Other Legal Considerations*).

- ☐ Facilitate management of finances by working closely with the individual your loved one has given power of attorney.

- ☐ Monitor your loved one's well-being, watching for signs of emotional, physical, and/or financial abuse.

- ☐ Alert family and caregivers to any problems.

Checklist: Signs you might need a geriatric care manager

- ☐ Your loved one has no family members nearby and you are trying to manage care from another state.

- ☐ You and/or your loved one are confused regarding housing arrangements as the disease progresses.

- ☐ The environment your loved one is currently living in is unsafe, but you do not know how to fix the situation.

- ☐ You and/or your family are burned out and unsure what care decisions would be best.

- ☐ You have been trying to research living arrangements, medical needs, and other care-related elements for Alzheimer's disease, but you are confused and frustrated.

- ☐ You are having difficulty communicating your loved one's needs to the facility where they are currently living.

- ☐ Your relationship with the facility where your loved one is currently living has become hostile and/or increasingly strained.

- ☐ Your family disagrees about the best course of action regarding care decisions and living arrangements.

- ☐ You and/or your loved one have many questions regarding financial and legal matters.

- ☐ Your loved one is in need of a strong care advocate.

- ☐ You and/or your family feel they would benefit from further education about changes that will need to be made as your loved one's disease progresses.

- [ ] Your loved one has become violent and/or withdrawn and depressed.

Checklist: What to look for when hiring a geriatric care manager

Geriatric Care Management Company:

- [ ] How long has the company been providing this service?
- [ ] Are the care managers trained to work with individuals who have Alzheimer's disease?
- [ ] What kind of training do they receive?
- [ ] Will the company provide references for the care manager?
- [ ] Do all employees undergo a background check?
- [ ] What types of backgrounds do their geriatric care managers have (e.g. social work, nursing, or counseling)?
- [ ] How does the company supervise their care managers?
- [ ] How often will you be updated about your loved one's situation?
- [ ] How much do they charge for a consultation?
- [ ] How much do they charge for services?
- [ ] Do they offer sliding scale fees?
- [ ] Do they offer the services you need most?
- [ ] Can they show you an example of a care plan they have used for a client with Alzheimer's disease?
- [ ] Are care managers available on weekends and holidays?

Independent Geriatric Care Managers:

- [ ] How long has the individual been offering geriatric care management services?

- [ ] How many clients has the individual worked with to date?

- [ ] Have any of these clients had Alzheimer's disease? If so, how many?

- [ ] Has the individual had training to work with individuals with Alzheimer's disease?

- [ ] Will the individual submit to a background check?

- [ ] Will the individual provide a list of references?

- [ ] What is the person's background (e.g., nursing, social work, or counseling)?

- [ ] Is the individual a certified geriatric care manager?

- [ ] Is the person familiar with the resources and overall area in which your loved one lives?

- [ ] How often will you be updated on your loved one's case?

- [ ] How much does the individual charge for services?

- [ ] How many other clients will the person have in addition to your loved one? Or will your loved one be the person's primary client?

- [ ] Is the individual friendly and approachable?

- [ ] Do you like the person? Do you think you could trust and work with this person long term?

- [ ] Does the individual seem responsible? Has the person answered your phone calls and/or emails in a timely manner?

- ☐ Can the individual provide examples of care plans that he or she has drawn up for other clients with Alzheimer's disease?

- ☐ Does the person offer the services you need most?

- ☐ Is the person in contact with an elder care attorney? Or does the person have a strong knowledge of elder care laws?

- ☐ Is the individual available for emergencies?

- ☐ Does the person provide consultation on weekends and holidays, if necessary?

- ☐ Does the person belong to any professional organizations in their field?

Leaving Home

When your loved one is first diagnosed with Alzheimer's disease, they will likely stay at home. A time will come, however, when you will notice the worsening of your loved one's condition. You will become aware of greater difficulties and dangerous situations your loved one is experiencing. You may even find it almost impossible to relax or sleep through the night because you are constantly worried about your loved one's safety. These are all signs that you should reassess your loved one's living situation. The following checklist highlights some signs that, either individually or in combination, could point to it no longer being safe for your loved one to live alone.

Checklist: Signs it is no longer safe for your loved one to live alone

- ☐ Your loved one has experienced a few instances of wandering.

- ☐ Your loved one has presented fire safety concerns, such as trying to cook but leaving the stove on or ignoring the smoke detectors.

- ☐ Your loved one gets confused or scared easily in their own house.

- ☐ Your loved one needs someone around 24 hours a day.

- ☐ Your loved one is scared to be alone.

- ☐ Your loved one is having difficulty successfully bathing or dressing.

- ☐ Your loved one has had a few minor falls and/or a more severe fall that caused injuries.

- ☐ Your loved one is becoming increasingly withdrawn and/or depressed.

- ☐ Weight loss has become apparent because your loved one has stopped eating.

- ☐ Your loved one frequently appears restless.

- ☐ Your loved one's ability to communicate has begun declining rapidly.

- ☐ Your loved one's hygiene difficulties have become apparent, such as not bathing, forgetting to brush teeth or hair, and wearing the same clothes each day.

- ☐ Your loved one has stopped taking medications properly.

- ☐ You feel that your loved one would not know what to do in case of an emergency, such as a fire, power outage, injury, or illness.

Chapter 2:
Moving in with a Caregiver

One option to consider when your loved one's condition progresses is for them to move in with a caregiver or to have a caregiver move into your loved one's home. Caregivers are usually children or close relatives of the individual with Alzheimer's disease. If you choose this option and become your loved one's caregiver, you need to consider home healthcare services, adult day care, routine changes, and safety concerns. As your loved one's needs progress, these factors may become more pronounced.

You may have difficulty knowing when your loved one can no longer live at home alone. However, it can be more difficult to know when your loved one should move in with a

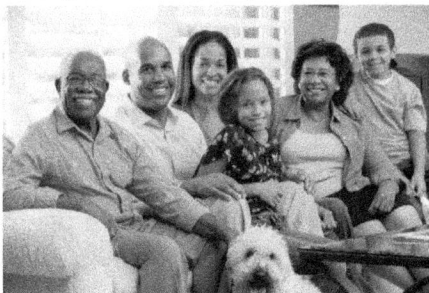

Credit: Monkey Business Images

caregiver—especially if that caregiver is you. When your loved one's condition progresses to a point where they must leave their home, you have several options. The first one many people consider is having their loved one move in with them. This is not the correct option for some, but for others it works well. You need to find the option that works best for you and your family. Consider the checklists below to determine if having your loved one move in with you is a good option.

Checklist: Should my loved one move in with me?

☐   Can my loved one safely live alone?

- [ ] Do I have extra room in my house for my loved one?

- [ ] Do I have the monetary resources to hire someone to be with my loved one during the day, or can I be home during the day with my loved one?

- [ ] Is this option more affordable than a live-in facility?

- [ ] Can I handle the emotional stress?

- [ ] Can my children/spouse handle the emotional stress?

- [ ] Will my job situation allow for me to leave at a moment's notice to take care of emergencies that will inevitably occur while my loved one lives at home?

- [ ] Have my loved one and I decided this should be the next step before considering an independent or full-time living facility?

- [ ] Do I have relief care options in place to avoid becoming burned out?

- [ ] Do I want full control over the care my loved one receives?

- [ ] Would I feel safer if my loved one was not living at home alone?

- [ ] Do my loved one and I get along well with one another? If you and your loved one do not communicate well in low-stress situations, then it is likely that having them move in with you will create unnecessary stress for both of you.

- [ ] Can I be patient with my loved one when they get frustrated or have a bad day?

- [ ] Is my loved one violent?

- ☐ Can my home be easily (and affordably) converted to meet the progressive needs of my loved one?

- ☐ Does my loved one need around-the-clock, skilled medical attention?

- ☐ Can my loved one eat on their own?

Checklist: Pros and cons of moving in with a caregiver

Pros:

- ☐ It is less expensive than a residential facility.

- ☐ Your loved one is close by.

- ☐ Your loved one will be in a familiar environment.

- ☐ You will be able to easily spend more time with your loved one.

- ☐ You will have more control over the type of care being received.

- ☐ You will be more involved with your loved one's medical care.

- ☐ You can ensure your loved one is getting daily exercise and cognitive stimulation.

- ☐ You will have more control over the visitors your loved one receives.

- ☐ You will be able to monitor for fraud and scams more easily.

Cons:

- ☐ Caregivers have a high chance of burnout.

- ☐ Caring for an individual who is losing their memory can be extremely stressful.

- ☐ Being a primary caregiver is time consuming.

- ☐ Your sleeping, eating, and daily habits will have to change to accommodate your loved one's habits.

- ☐ Your daily routines could be disrupted, particularly if you have young children.

- ☐ You will be responsible for your loved one's safety and well-being.

- ☐ As the disease progresses, it may become more difficult to be the primary caregiver.

- ☐ Your loved one may eventually have to be moved to a residential facility.

- ☐ You will need to hire home healthcare services.

Before deciding to have your loved one move in with you and your family, you should know the duties and responsibilities you will have. Live-in caregivers to individuals with Alzheimer's disease often become burned out because they do not understand the amount of work, and sometimes stress, that comes with this role. For example, in the United States, more than 16 million people provide an estimated 18.5 billion hours of unpaid care to individuals with Alzheimer's disease or other dementias. Collectively, this care is valued at approximately $234 billion. Therefore, taking on the role of live-in caregiver is a momentous decision. The following checklist discusses some of the responsibilities you will have if your loved one moves into your home.

Checklist: What are the roles of a live-in caregiver?

- ☐ Implement a daily routine.

- ☐ Plan nutritious, healthy meals.

- ☐ Prepare medications and monitor if they are taken correctly.

- ☐ Watch for signs of adverse reactions to medications.

- ☐ Organize daily physical activities and exercise, if possible.

- ☐ Organize daily activities to engage the mind.

- ☐ Ensure your loved one has opportunities for socializing.

- ☐ Plan various activities to keep your loved one from sitting around most of the day.

- ☐ Organize your loved one's participation in spiritual activities, if this is something they have always done or they want to do.

- ☐ Plan visits with family and friends.

- ☐ Monitor holiday celebrations, and your loved one's reaction to these events, to prevent anxiety and stress.

- ☐ Support your loved one when they become discouraged, frustrated, or anxious.

- ☐ Prevent your loved one from experiencing too much stress. (High stress will speed progression of the disease and cause unnecessary anxiety.)

- ☐ Assist your loved one with bathing, dressing, and toileting when needed.

- ☐ Help your loved one with daily grooming, such as brushing their teeth, cleaning their dentures, shaving, cleaning their fingernails, etc.

- ☐ Stay patient and calm when helping your loved one.

- ☐ Work to ensure your loved one's safety in the home, as well as out in public.

- ☐ Assess and modify the house for safety as your loved one's illness progresses.

- ☐ Watch for signs of wandering and sundowning (increased confusion and disorientation that generally occurs in the late afternoon or early evening).

- ☐ Prevent your loved one from wandering, especially at night when you could be sleeping.

- ☐ Ensure that your loved one is getting enough sleep.

- ☐ Arrange doctor and specialist appointments.

- ☐ Arrange and/or provide transportation to appointments.

- ☐ Act as an advocate for your loved one with doctors, and potentially even other family members. (This is primarily the responsibility of a healthcare agent.)

- ☐ Monitor your loved one for signs of advancing cognitive deterioration.

- ☐ Watch for significant changes in your loved one's personality and/or communication skills.

- ☐ Manage, or help manage, your loved one's finances. (This is primarily the responsibility of a durable power of attorney for finances.)

- ☐ Hire home services (home healthcare, homemaker, and/or companion services) when they are needed.

- ☐ For more information about responsibilities associated with being a live-in caregiver, see *Caregiver Resources for Helping with Activities of Daily Living*.

If you have made the decision to have your loved one move in with you, this will likely be a difficult time for your loved one. They will be leaving their home, which will greatly decrease their independence. Moving in with an adult child or relative on top of that may seem to your loved one as though they are no longer trusted or able to provide their own care. Maintaining independence is important when your loved one moves in with you, because increased independence can be beneficial to their overall well-being. The checklist below discusses some tips for helping your loved one maintain their independence after the move.

Checklist: Tips for maintaining independence when living with a caregiver

- ☐ Encourage your loved one to help around the house with small tasks such as setting the table, washing dishes, folding laundry, etc.

- ☐ Have your loved one help you prepare a meal they used to cook regularly.

- ☐ Ask your loved one to help with the baking, if that is something they once enjoyed.

- ☐ Ask for their opinion on cooking; maybe have them taste the food and offer suggestions. (Note: As the disease progresses, your loved one may begin to lose their sense of smell and taste.)

- ☐ Try not to be overprotective and do everything for your loved one. They can likely still help out in many ways.

- ☐ If your loved one is having difficulty performing a particular task, offer to help but do not take over or do the task for them.

- ☐ Make sure to give your loved one choices. If they become anxious due to having too many options, limit choices to two things. For example, ask your loved one if they would like meatloaf or soup for dinner.

- ☐ If you have children, encourage your loved one to help with them. Being around children can be a low-stress situation for individuals with

Alzheimer's disease because they are less likely to feel as though they are being judged. It could also help bring back good memories of your loved one's childhood.

☐ Ask your loved one to help care for your pet (if you have one). Your loved one could help take the pet for walks (with someone's company if they are prone to wandering) or help feed the animal. Pets can be very therapeutic.

☐ Encourage your loved one to help you with gardening or taking care of indoor plants, if that was something they once enjoyed. Ensure that none of the plants are poisonous if ingested, and always stay with your loved when using tools in the garden that could lead to injury.

☐ Plan outings once a week if your loved one is able, and give them a choice of the location.

☐ If your loved one has stopped participating in hobbies or activities because the illness has made it difficult, offer to participate in those activities together. For example, you could go for walks together or work on a craft they enjoy.

☐ Give your loved one as much freedom in the house as possible.

☐ If your loved one has started to have incontinence problems, do not make a big deal out of it. Buy disposable underwear and leave them in the bathroom your loved one uses; tell your loved one where you placed the underwear, but do not mention it again unless necessary.

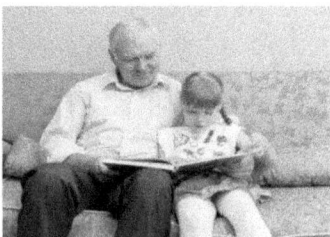

Credit: Sergey Nivens

☐ Encourage your loved one to participate in decisions about their health, activities, and options whenever possible.

Caregiver Agreements

When your loved one is unable to provide their own care, a family member often steps in to become a caregiver. Sometimes, the caregiver goes to your loved one's home for several hours each day to provide care. In other situations, the caregiver may move in with your loved one or your loved one may move in with the caregiver, as discussed above. This can create both a financial and emotional hardship for the caregiver, especially if the caregiver is required to give up a steady job with benefits to provide care. If one individual is providing the majority of care for your loved one, your family may want to create a caregiver agreement that allows your loved one to pay the caregiver for the care they provide. The following checklists provide basic information about caregiver agreements as well as information that should be included in the caregiver agreement. For sample care agreements, see the links in the Resources.

Checklist: Basics about a caregiver agreement

☐ A caregiver agreement is a contract between an ill individual and a caregiver to list caregiving responsibilities and compensation for care provided.

☐ A caregiver agreement can also be called a personal care agreement, long-term care personal support services agreement, elder care contract, family care contract, or caregiver contract.

☐ A caregiver agreement can be used to compensate a family member who has made a great personal sacrifice in order to provide care for a loved one.

This prevents the caregiver from experiencing undue financial hardships due to their caregiving responsibilities.

☐ The caregiver agreement should be put in writing. This allows the caregiver and family members to have a record of the caregiver's responsibilities and compensation as well as provide proof to Medicaid and other government assistance programs that the transfer of money between your loved one and the caregiver was for caregiving services and not a gift. (See *Long-Term Care Insurance, Power of Attorney, Wealth Management, and Other First Steps* for more information about Medicaid eligibility and gifts.)

☐ A caregiving agreement can help avoid family conflicts over who should provide care and what type of care they should provide.

☐ Because a caregiving agreement may affect the inheritance, all family members should help construct the caregiving agreement, especially the amount the caregiver will be compensated.

☐ A caregiver agreement is used to stipulate payment for future caregiving services. It should not provide compensation for past caregiving serviced.

☐ A caregiver agreement provides your loved one with peace of mind that they will be cared for when they are no longer able to provide their own care.

☐ A lawyer is not needed to complete the caregiver agreement, but it may be beneficial to consult a lawyer for complicated agreements.

Checklist: Characteristics of a caregiver

☐ Often an adult child of the individual with Alzheimer's disease, although adult grandchildren, other relatives, or friends may also provide care

- ☐ Should live close to your loved one with Alzheimer's disease

- ☐ Should be someone your loved one knows, not a stranger

- ☐ Often has few personal responsibilities, such as no minor children living at home

- ☐ Should be willing to give up a paying job if necessary to care for your loved one, provided they will be paid for providing care to your loved one

- ☐ Willing to take on the enormous time commitment and responsibility needed to care for a loved one with Alzheimer's disease

- ☐ Responsible and even-tempered

- ☐ Understands the list of responsibilities as well as how to perform the needed tasks

Checklist: Information to include in a caregiver agreement

- ☐ The date care should begin. For individuals with Alzheimer's disease, this may be a vague date in the future based on the progression of the disease.

- ☐ How long the agreement is in effect (e.g., one year, five years, for the lifetime of the ill individual).

- ☐ A detailed description of care to be provided. You may want to have a care assessment conducted in the home or consult your loved one's medical records to help determine the care needed. Specifically defining the care tasks to be completed and the time they will take will help compensation and time expectations be more reasonable.

- ☐ Provisions for expanded care responsibilities as your loved one's disease progresses.

- [ ] Where the care will take place (e.g., at the loved one's home, in the caregiver's home). Allow for a change of location as needed based on your loved one's stage of disease.

- [ ] How many hours of caregiving will be provided each week. For individuals with Alzheimer's disease, the number of caregiving hours may need to be given on a sliding scale based on the progression of the disease. Language should allow for flexibility, such as "up to 20 hours per week" or "no less than 160 hours per month."

- [ ] The amount of compensation for the caregiver. Compensation for care should be similar to what the family would pay a third party to provide care. The family may need to do some research into the amount they would pay a caregiving service for a similar level of care. The amount of compensation should reflect the complexity of caregiving duties and the time spent on caregiving duties.

- [ ] When the caregiver will be compensated (e.g., weekly, bi-weekly, monthly).

- [ ] Provisions for raises in the future to compensate for a job well done.

- [ ] Provisions for living expense compensation (e.g., room and board, utilities) if your loved one lives with the caregiver; also make sure that homeowners insurance covers liabilities such as work injuries.

- [ ] Provisions for health insurance and other benefits for the caregiver, especially if they resigned from a job with benefits to provide care for your loved one.

- [ ] Your loved one's responsibility vs. the caregiver's responsibility for paying withholding taxes and Social Security.

- ☐ Provisions for incidental out-of-pocket expenses, including but not limited to home modifications for safety.

- ☐ Determine who will write the checks. This should be the power of attorney for finances; if the caregiver is the power of attorney, consult a trustee or other legal representative.

- ☐ If the caregiver will be responsible for transportation, stipulate the level of car insurance that is needed.

- ☐ Provisions for respite time or vacation time for the caregiver.

- ☐ Provisions for caregiving backup if the caregiver goes on vacation, gets sick, or needs respite time.

- ☐ A statement that the agreement can be modified only by mutual agreement by both parties. Any modifications should be put in writing and signed and dated by both parties.

- ☐ A statement that the caregiver can void the contract if the caregiving duties exceed their abilities. For example, a caregiver may feel unqualified to care for your loved one in the final stages of Alzheimer's disease.

- ☐ Signatures of both parties and the date. If your loved one is not legally competent to sign the document, their durable power of attorney for finances or conservator can sign for them. If the caregiver and your loved one's legal financial representative are the same person, consider consulting an attorney.

Checklist: Types of caregiver duties listed in a caregiver agreement

- ☐ Hygiene care (e.g., bathing, dressing, grooming)
- ☐ Nutrition (e.g., cooking, special diet considerations, feeding, grocery shopping)
- ☐ Mobility (e.g., assisting with transfers from the bed to a chair)
- ☐ Monitoring medications
- ☐ Tracking changes in health
- ☐ Companionship
- ☐ Monitoring for safety (e.g., wandering, driving, home safety, medication safety)
- ☐ Housekeeping (e.g., cleaning, laundry, dishes, errands); may list individual tasks if needed
- ☐ Outdoor maintenance (e.g., mowing lawn, trimming bushes, raking leaves, snow removal)
- ☐ Finances (e.g., paying household bills, paying medical bills, balancing the checkbook); note that this may be the duty of a power of attorney rather than the caregiver
- ☐ Car maintenance (e.g., taking your loved one's car to the shop for oil changes)
- ☐ Transportation to appointments and events; consider mileage in compensation
- ☐ Consulting with physicians and other medical personnel; note that this may be the duty of a healthcare agent rather than the caregiver
- ☐ Creating a daily log of activities; this will help with Medicare or other documentation as well as provide evidence of services provided

□   Recording payment of expenses for government assistance documentation

Caregiver Burnout

If you are your loved one's primary caregiver, you may suffer the effects of caregiver burnout over time. Caregiver burnout occurs due to an accumulation of stress and responsibility that the caregiver experiences. If your loved one moves in with you, a routine will likely develop. However, as the disease progresses into the middle and later stages, this routine will probably become more and more complicated, which will ultimately leave you with more responsibility and less time for yourself. The signs of caregiver burnout are gradual, but you need to watch for them in order to avoid later complications. Being aware of the signs will also enable you to work toward reversing the effects. The following checklist discusses the signs of caregiver burnout.

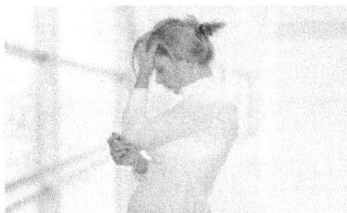

Credit: Piotr Marcinski

Checklist: Signs of caregiver burnout

□   You feel more overwhelmed than usual.

□   You do not exercise or relax because you feel that there is no time.

□   Your anxiety levels have started increasing.

□   You have lost your temper with a loved one because they are not responding the way you want or expect.

□   You are yelling at and/or becoming angry with coworkers, loved ones, and friends for no reason.

- [ ] Your emotions change quickly and drastically (e.g., you are angry one minute and extremely sad the next).

- [ ] You are not sleeping well due to stress or anxiety.

- [ ] You find that you are exhausted all the time.

- [ ] You are frequently giving up social and family events.

- [ ] You have not spent time with friends or participated in enjoyable activities in months.

- [ ] You no longer enjoy activities you once favored.

- [ ] You feel that you are unable to give your loved one the help they need.

- [ ] Your weight or appetite has changed.

- [ ] You have been ill more often than usual.

- [ ] You are having trouble concentrating on tasks.

- [ ] You are having difficulty remembering appointments or events.

- [ ] You have had thoughts of suicide.

- [ ] You have had thoughts about hurting your loved one.

- [ ] You find yourself wishing it would all be over so that your stress could end.

If you think you might be suffering from caregiver burnout, seek help for yourself and assistance with your caregiving responsibilities. Numerous support groups exist where you can meet with other people in your area who are experiencing similar difficulties. (Please see the Resources for help finding support groups near you.) If you need a break from caregiver duties, consider taking a short vacation or having family members or a service come in one or two afternoons a week to give you time for yourself. The checklist below discusses some options for services that could help give you a break from your caregiver duties.

Checklist: Respite care and adult day care

Respite Care:

- ☐ Respite care provides you with a few hours to get out of the house and have some time to yourself.

- ☐ It occurs in your home, so your loved one would not have to leave.

- ☐ It gives your loved one a chance to interact with another person.

- ☐ It can offer you extra time to do errands.

- ☐ It helps prevent caregiver burnout.

- ☐ Friends, family, or neighbors can provide respite care.

- ☐ Community organizations offer respite care services.

- ☐ You can hire services such as homemaker and companion services to provide respite care (see Home Services).

- ☐ Some residential facilities offer short-term stays for respite care (one night to a few weeks).

Adult Day Care:

- ☐ Adult day care is a place where your loved one is cared for by trained staff while you are at work, running errands, or taking a needed break.

- ☐ You will be able to relax knowing that your loved one is safe and cared for.

- ☐ Transportation is sometimes provided to and from the day care facility.

- [ ] Adult day care is offered in a location outside of your home.

- [ ] Most centers are open between seven and ten hours a day.

- [ ] Some facilities are open over the weekend and have evening hours.

- [ ] Most centers have social workers and nurses on staff.

- [ ] The staff is often trained to work with individuals who have dementia. Some adult day centers specialize in providing care for individuals with Alzheimer's disease.

- [ ] These facilities supply nutritious meals and snacks throughout the day.

- [ ] You loved one can receive assistance with eating, when necessary.

- [ ] You loved one is provided with assistance taking medications during the day.

- [ ] Your loved one will engage in light physical exercise.

- [ ] Physical, occupational, and speech therapy are generally offered at these facilities.

- [ ] These facilities often teach relaxation techniques.

- [ ] Many facilities offer pet therapy and music therapy, both of which can be very beneficial.

- [ ] Your loved one is provided with activities to stimulate their mind.

- [ ] Your loved one will be able to interact with others and engage in social activities.

- Activities such as games, gardening, field trips, and crafts are planned throughout the day to keep your loved one entertained and active.

- Some facilities offer counseling for both your loved one and your family, if needed.

- Medicaid generally covers most, if not all, adult day care costs.

- Private insurance and long-term care insurance will sometimes cover the cost of adult day care.

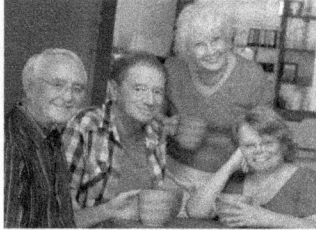

Credit: Creatista

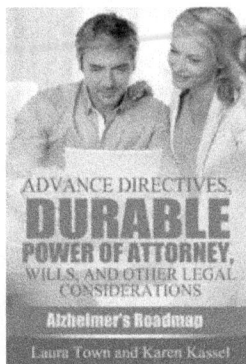

Chapter 3:
Moving to Assisted Living

Because of the immeasurable stress placed on the caregiver and the potential for caregiver burnout, having your loved one live at home alone or with a caregiver is often not preferable when your loved one is in the later stages of the disease. If you decide that having your loved one move in with you is not a

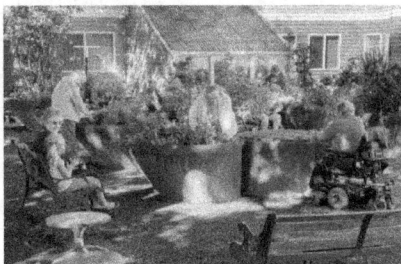

Credit: Jamie Hooper

good decision for you and your family, consider an independent facility. Independent facilities are also referred to as assisted living facilities, adult living centers, and supported care facilities. These residences allow those living there to have a greater sense of independence than they would experience in a hospital or nursing home, but the facility also provides assistance with day-to-day activities.

When Dad reached the middle stages of the disease, we had a caregiver there with him for 12 hours each day, and that worked for a few weeks until he started wandering at night. We then had to have caregivers there with him for 24 hours a day. We were blessed that dad's long-term care insurance covered it. However, the costs quickly began depleting his policy. After a year or so, we determined that we had to move him to assisted living at half the cost of 24 hour care so we could keep a strong reserve in his policy to cover him for more years. This was a very hard move, but it was the right move. At first, Dad was angry and unhappy. He hated leaving his home. He became depressed. The first month was difficult. But after the first month, he had several good months.

Moving your loved one to an independent care facility such as an assisted living facility can be a tough decision for all involved. You generally would take this step either when your loved one can no longer live alone or when your loved one becomes too progressed in the disease for a caregiver to offer everything your loved one needs. Independent facilities do not offer around-the-clock skilled medical care. If this is needed, then you should consider a nursing home or other full-time care facility. The following checklist details some signs that your loved one, or you as their caregiver, might want to consider moving your loved one to an independent living facility.

Checklist: Signs an independent living facility could be beneficial

Your Loved One:

- ☐ Has started wandering often.

- ☐ Has become lost due to wandering.

- ☐ Has been brought home by police and/or neighbors because they were wandering and became disoriented.

- ☐ Has recently become more isolated, even depressed at times.

- ☐ Experiences little to no socialization during the day.

- ☐ Falls often.

- ☐ Becomes more and more confused on a daily basis.

- ☐ Has experienced difficulty cooking.

- ☐ Becomes violent (physically or verbally) or acts out frequently.

- ☐ Has started sundowning.

- ☐ Is not safe in their current living environment due to increasing symptoms of the disease; however, the person can still perform the activities of daily living independently or with minimal help.

The Caregiver:

- ☐ Has begun losing sleep due to worrying about a loved one.

- ☐ Experiences extreme anger, sadness, and/or aggression because of stress and/or caregiver duties.

- ☐ Loses patience with their loved one often.

- ☐ Consistently gives up social or work events.

- ☐ Does not have time alone to rest and recuperate.

- ☐ Loses or gains weight due to stress.

- ☐ Experiences health problems.

- ☐ Has begun drinking alcohol, using drugs, or smoking to deal with stress.

- ☐ Can no longer keep up with their caregiver duties.

- ☐ Constantly worries that their loved one will be injured due to escalating symptoms.

- ☐ Cannot physically help their loved one up if the individual falls.

- ☐ Has begun to resent their loved one for being ill.

The services that independent living facilities provide depend on the individual facility, and particularly on whether it specializes in memory care. However, the following checklist highlights some of the services these facilities often provide.

Checklist: Services independent facilities often provide

- ☐ Housing, either individual apartments, suites, or shared rooms.

- ☐ Housekeeping services.

- ☐ Laundry services.

- ☐ Three meals a day, often provided in a group setting; however, most facilities will allow residents to dine alone in their rooms if they want to.

- ☐ Assistance with eating, such as if food needs to be cut into smaller pieces.

- ☐ 24-hour staff for assistance with any needs that may arise.

- ☐ Recreational activities and events.

- ☐ Therapeutic activities, such as music therapy and pet therapy.

- ☐ Activities to encourage exercise.

- ☐ Relaxation activities such as yoga and meditation.

- ☐ Help with bathing, dressing, and toileting as needed.

- ☐ Assistance with medications, including both reminding residents when to take medications and what dose of medication to take.

- ☐ 24-hour monitoring of the facility to prevent residents from wandering.

- ☐ Emergency call systems in all rooms.

- ☐ 24-hour security around the facility.

- ☐ Counseling and therapy services.

- ☐ Physical and speech therapy.

- ☐ Transportation to doctor's appointments.

- ☐ Barber and beautician services for residents.

- ☐ Limited health services.

- ☐ Consultations from a nutritionist when needed.

- ☐ Frequent visits from a nurse on staff to ensure the resident is doing well.

Before choosing an independent facility, you and your loved one, if possible, should visit the place multiple times to get a feel for the atmosphere. You should also do research into the services that facility offers as well as their individual policies. Consider the following checklist of what to look for in an independent care facility.

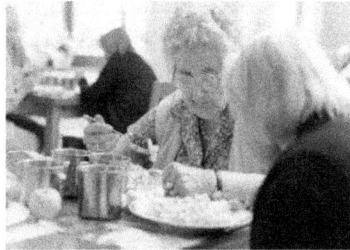

Credit: Kristo-Gothard Hunor

Checklist: Questions to consider when looking for an independent living facility

- ☐ Do they have a special unit/facility for those with Alzheimer's disease?

- ☐ Do they accept residents in the early stages of Alzheimer's disease?

- ☐ What behaviors will result in a resident being asked to leave?

- ☐ Will residents who progress into a later stage of Alzheimer's disease need to move out, or does the facility have the ability to care for them?

- [ ] Do they offer hospice services if needed? Or will the person need to be transferred to a nursing home?

- [ ] What kind of training does their staff have in caring for residents with dementia/Alzheimer's disease?

- [ ] Do they offer any activities specifically geared toward memory retention?

- [ ] Do residents have single apartments or will they share with others?

- [ ] How many residents are normally in a living area together?

- [ ] What is the ratio of staff to residents?

- [ ] How often do nurses check on residents?

- [ ] Do they accept residents in wheelchairs?

- [ ] Do they accept residents with oxygen tanks?

- [ ] Do common rooms, activity centers, offices, etc. all look the same, or do they have distinct design features to help eliminate confusion?

- [ ] Are there options for prepared foods if residents decide they do not want to cook?

- [ ] Are the grounds and rooms of the facility maintained well? Or are they run down and dirty?

- [ ] What are the outdoor areas of the facility like? Is the facility near a busy street? Are there paths for walking?

- [ ] Is there a gate or barrier of some sort around the facility to dissuade wandering?

- [ ] Is the staff friendly and receptive when you visit?

- [ ] Are the staff members outgoing?

- [ ] Do the other residents at the facility look happy?

- [ ] Can you visit your loved one at any time? Or are there visiting hours?

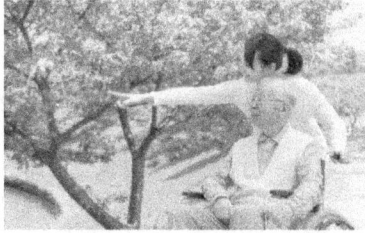
Credit: Mykeyruna

- [ ] Do they provide outings for the residents to local stores or attractions? If so, how often do these outings happen?

- [ ] What is the supervision like on the outings? If your loved one gets confused and wanders, will there be enough staff to notice your loved one is no longer with the group?

- [ ] Does the facility accept your loved one's insurance plan?

- [ ] What extra costs are included at the facility that are not generally covered by insurance? For example, some activities or programs are not covered by insurance.

- [ ] Does the facility have any citations against them currently?

- [ ] Has the facility had any citations in the past? If so, how serious were the citations and how long ago did they occur?

- [ ] What is the facility's policy regarding medication? Do they hand out medication daily to residents? Or are residents expected to keep their own medications?

- [ ] What is the facility's policy in the case of a medical emergency?

- [ ] Does each apartment have an emergency response system to easily call for help?

- [ ] What is the staff coverage/assistance like on the weekends and holidays?

Independent living facilities are generally reserved for those who do not need skilled medical care but may require assistance in their day-to-day activities. As such, these facilities would be more appropriate if your loved one is in the earlier stages of Alzheimer's disease. When my dad was in assisted living, I was able to take him out to lunch once a week. He seemed to really enjoy these ventures outside the facility, and he loved the food. I often brought my young son with me, and it was a chance for Dad to really be able to act as a grandpa. All went well for five to six months. Then one day, I took dad to a new place that I thought he would like. The meal was perfect, Dad was actually conversing coherently, and we had a wonderful conversation. I dropped Dad off at his room in the assisted living facility and left feeling grateful for the day we had. An hour later, I received a call from the facility. Dad had hit someone. This was the first fight Dad was ever in. Completely unprovoked, Dad started punching people.

Dad had to be sent to a psychiatric facility. In meeting

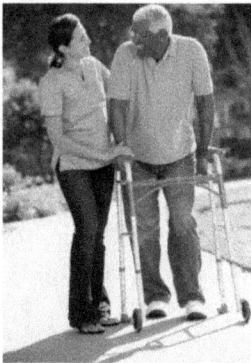

Credit: Monkey Business Images

with the geriatric psychiatrist, I was told that taking Dad out of his environment could be triggering these episodes. The psychiatrist followed him around for a day and didn't notice anything unusual. Dad went back to assisted living. He hit someone else. Rinse and repeat. In my state, the patient who has three psychiatric stays at a hospital can be denied entrance by any nursing home.

56

Dad was at two. If I wanted to have some choice in the home that I placed Dad in, I had to move fast. It was at this point that I knew I needed to move Dad into a full-time care facility.

Chapter 4:
Moving to a Full-Time
Care Facility

Full-time care facilities are generally either nursing homes or settings very similar to nursing homes that specialize in memory loss. If your loved one requires medical attention, 24-hour care, assistance with walking and dressing, and/or around-the-clock supervision, a full-time care facility could be helpful. These facilities employ teams of nurses, social workers, therapists, nutritionists, and doctors to aid residents in their day-to-day needs. In addition, most nursing homes have common areas where activities are held as well as options for communal dining so that residents can socialize with one another if they choose to.

After Dad's aggressive episodes at the assisted living facility, I knew I had to decide which full-time care facility I wanted to place him in. Dad was already on the waiting lists for the best nursing homes, but no spots were open. A nursing home with a "below average" rating was close to my home, so close that it was within walking distance. I talked to the geriatric psychiatrist and agonized over what to do. He told me, "Even if it was the Ritz Carlton, your dad would not know. You have to do what is best for you." I placed dad in the nursing home, and I wasn't happy. I'm still not happy with it. However, I also recognize that I would not be happy with any facility. Dad is safe and fed and not in any visible emotional distress or pain. Sometimes that is the best we can do.

Like me, many individuals view full-time care facilities, such as nursing homes, as either unnecessary or negative in some way. Due to this misconception, many caregivers and family members feel extreme guilt when a loved one with Alzheimer's disease is placed in a long-term care facility. The truth, however, is that your loved one will likely need some form of full-time care toward the later stages of their disease. The checklist below highlights some signs that your loved one might benefit from a long-term care facility.

Checklist: Signs your loved one could benefit from a long-term care facility

Your loved one:

- ☐ Has begun wandering during the day and at night.

- ☐ Has been injured due to wandering.

- ☐ Needs daily medical assistance from a professional.

- ☐ Has a serious medical condition in addition to Alzheimer's disease.

- ☐ Needs 24-hour care and supervision.

- ☐ Has begun aspirating or choking on their food regularly.

- ☐ Is now bedridden.

- ☐ Is incontinent and/or is using objects other than the toilet for voiding.

- ☐ Is becoming sexually, physically, or emotionally abusive.

- ☐ Has lost the ability to communicate their needs (through speech, hand gestures, or writing).

- ☐ Needs frequent assistance walking or standing.

- ☐ Is no longer safe in their environment.

- ☐ Requires pain management, medical care, and/or hospice care.

- ☐ Has symptoms that are becoming too much for their caregiver to manage.

☐   Needs physical assistance with eating.

☐   Requires daily management of medications.

The services provided by long-term care facilities will vary based on the type of institution. For example, specialized units called memory care units will have services geared toward individuals with Alzheimer's disease, whereas nursing homes will generally have fewer services available that work specifically with memory loss. Some nursing homes, however, do have units that specialize in Alzheimer's care. The following checklist discusses some of the services provided by full-time care facilities.

Checklist: Services provided at full-time care facilities

☐   Specialized medical care

☐   24-hour-a-day nursing services

☐   Assistance taking medications

☐   Prescribing new medications

☐   Wound care

☐   Preventative care and access to immunizations, such as flu and pneumonia vaccines

☐   Arrangements with local hospitals in case of a medical emergency

☐   Palliative care; some facilities will provide hospice services, but in many cases you will need to arrange this yourself if they allow it.

☐   Dental care; some facilities will provide monthly access to a dentist, but this is not the case in all areas so check with the individual facility.

☐   Health and nutrition management

- [ ] Three balanced meals a day, generally served in a dining room, but residents can request food to be served in their room.

- [ ] Help with any feeding needs

- [ ] Housekeeping

- [ ] Laundry

- [ ] Assistance bathing and dressing

- [ ] Monitoring and assistance with personal hygiene

- [ ] Assistance with toileting and the use of garments for incontinence

- [ ] Recreational activities with other residents

- [ ] Activities and programs to promote physical exercise

- [ ] Memory retention activities

- [ ] Religious and cultural programs and activities

- [ ] Physical therapy and speech therapy

- [ ] A secure environment with 24-hour-a-day monitoring

- [ ] Management of behavior changes and outbursts.

- [ ] Design features organized so as not to be visually distracting or confusing; for example, all the hallways and offices will not look the same.

- [ ] Large, descriptive signs labeling offices, bathrooms, dining rooms, and resident quarters to help in identification and the reduction of confusion

When deciding on a full-time care facility, you should visit the facility at different parts of the day and week to see how the staff interacts with residents, how activities such as meal times are conducted, and how the environment changes with different staff and activities. For example, visit the facility both in the morning and at meal times to see how much the noise volume increases. You can also visit your state's website to check how the home is rated overall for service and quality. The following checklist highlights some areas to pay particular attention to when deciding on a long-term care facility.

Checklist: Questions to consider when looking for a full-time care facility

- ☐ Do they admit those with Alzheimer's disease?

- ☐ Do they have a special Alzheimer's disease unit? If so, how is it different than the other units?

- ☐ Can those who progress to the later stages of Alzheimer's disease stay at the facility, or do they have to move?

- ☐ Is the staff trained to work with patients with Alzheimer's disease?

- ☐ Will they provide you with a sample care plan for a resident who has Alzheimer's disease?

- ☐ Do they provide any activities aimed at those with memory loss?

- ☐ Does the facility perform background checks on all employees? What are their hiring restrictions in accordance with these background checks? In other words, if a person has ever been suspected of abuse or mistreatment, will the facility still hire them?

- ☐ What is their policy for a staff member who uses physical force against a resident? It should be zero-tolerance.

- ☐ What kind of security is in place if a resident wanders or becomes confused?

- ☐ Where are the cameras at the facility located? Will you be able to have access to the footage if needed (such as in cases of suspected abuse)?

- ☐ Do they have activities available every day?

- ☐ How much social interaction do residents have with staff and one another?

- ☐ Do residents share rooms with one another, or are there single rooms available?

- ☐ Is there an outside area for residents?

- ☐ How are meal times handled?

- ☐ How many people are available to help the resident eat? Patients cannot use silverware at some stages of the disease.

- ☐ Can residents eat in their rooms if they wish?

- ☐ How does the staff promote and/or monitor healthy nutrition?

- ☐ What forms of nutritional assessment will be conducted? How often will these assessments be conducted?

- ☐ Are families encouraged to participate in activities, meal times, and overall care?

- ☐ How are medications stored? (They should be locked and far away from residents.)

- ☐ Do the residents at the facility appear to be happy?

- ☐ Are the current residents well-groomed and dressed appropriately?

- ☐ Is the staff friendly and respectful?

- ☐ Is the setup/design of the facility easy to navigate?

- ☐ What are the visiting hours? Do those hours work with your schedule?

- ☐ What is the ratio of nurses and doctors to residents?

- ☐ What is the ratio of social workers to residents?

- ☐ What is the ration of nurses (RNs) to staff/CNAs to staff on the days and on the weekends?

- ☐ What is the employee turnover rate?

- ☐ What policies are in place in the case of a medical emergency?

- ☐ Do they provide hospice services if they are needed?

- ☐ Can your loved one's living space be decorated in any way they choose?

- ☐ What religious and/or cultural services do they have in place for residents?

- ☐ What doctors will be caring for your loved one, and will you be able to meet and approve them before any care is given?

- ☐ What is the reputation of the facility?

- ☐ Does the facility currently have any citations pending against them? If so, how serious are the citations?

- ☐ Has the facility had citations in the past?

- ☐ Is the facility covered by your loved one's insurance provider?

- ☐ How long is the waiting list to get a bed at the facility? Will it be longer if your loved one is on Medicaid?

- [ ] How will you be billed for services? What extras should you expect on top of the monthly fee (i.e., haircuts, activities, incontinence, briefs, gloves)?

- [ ] Can you speak to current staff, residents, and the family members of residents before you choose the facility?

- [ ] How is the facility designed? Do all the hallways and common areas look the same? Or are there distinguishing features to prevent confusion?

- [ ] Is the facility overly noisy? What is the facility's policy on noise control?

- [ ] What types of activities are offered to residents? How frequently are activities held?

Memory Care Units

Some assisted living and long-term care facilities are specifically tailored to those with Alzheimer's disease and are called memory care units, special care units, or memory support programs. These units are generally set apart from the other areas of the facility and have dedicated staff. Short-term or long-term care facilities that offer specialized programs for individuals with Alzheimer's disease can be very beneficial for your loved one. Your loved one will be around others who have memory difficulties, and the staff will be trained to work with individuals who have dementia.

If you are unsure if a facility you are considering has a program for a loved one with Alzheimer's disease, you can always check their website to see if they have information there, or call the facility and ask. The following checklist details some of the features of memory care units.

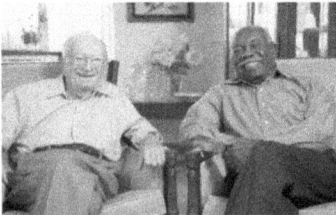

Credit: Monkey Business

Checklist: Features of memory care units

- [ ] All residents have either dementia or Alzheimer's disease.

- [ ] Staff has specialized training to care for those with dementia or Alzheimer's disease.

- [ ] Staff receives frequent training in order to stay knowledgeable about new research, findings, and changes to suggested care practices.

- [ ] Activities and games are aimed at memory retention.

- [ ] Enhanced safety protocols are in place.

- [ ] Large signs and other measures are in place to help decrease disorientation and confusion.

- [ ] The facility often provides a higher degree of individualized attention.

- [ ] The facility features private or semi-private living areas.

- [ ] Rooms are designed to promote resident independence.

- [ ] Both nurses and social workers provide 24-hour supervision and care.

- [ ] The ratio of nurses and doctors to residents is high to provide specialized and dedicated care.

- [ ] More pet, music, art, and relaxation therapies are available.

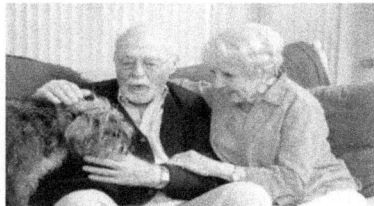

Credit: Lisa F. Young

- ☐ Personalized programs are tailored to help individual residents.

- ☐ A larger emphasis is placed on recreational and social activities to promote stimulation and avoid sedentary activities.

Memory care units are designed specifically for individuals with Alzheimer's disease or other forms of dementia. As such, a facility like this would be an ideal place for your loved one to live if you can find one in your area that is covered by your loved one's insurance or is otherwise affordable.

Psychiatric Facilities

If your loved one develops problems with aggression or violence, they may be placed in a psychiatric facility, especially if they were in an assisted living or long-term care facility and injured a caregiver or another resident. Care facilities must protect their workers and residents, and having a resident who is a danger to others is a liability many facilities will not tolerate. If you are unable to handle the care of your loved one outside of a long-term care facility, your loved one may be placed in a psychiatric facility and held involuntarily until the situation subsides. To understand more about psychiatric facilities, see the checklists below.

Checklist: Reasons your loved one may be placed in a psychiatric facility

- ☐ Biting
- ☐ Hitting
- ☐ Pushing
- ☐ Cussing
- ☐ Pulling hair

- [ ] Delusions
- [ ] Paranoia
- [ ] Hallucinations
- [ ] Fighting
- [ ] Threatening someone with a sharp object
- [ ] Spitting
- [ ] Mood swings
- [ ] Threatening to commit suicide
- [ ] Yelling
- [ ] Stomping on someone

Checklist: What to expect from a psychiatric facility

- [ ] Your loved one may be held for 72 hours or more without your approval. An emergency hospitalization for evaluation, also called a psychiatric hold or pick-up, is typically for a fixed period such as 72 hours, but the law for this varies by state.

- [ ] Your loved one should be assessed by a physician.

- [ ] The physician will likely try different combinations of medications to control aggressive or psychiatric symptoms.

- [ ] The physician will likely try to identify triggers for psychiatric or aggressive behavior. For individuals with Alzheimer's disease, seemingly unlikely triggers can cause aggression, such as a change in environment, asking your loved one to change clothing, or trying to force them to take medication or take a bath.

- [ ] Your loved one may be placed in a solitary room.

- ☐ Your loved one may be restrained by the arms and/or legs.

- ☐ Your loved one's health and mental acuity may decline rapidly after a stay in a psychiatric facility, or it may improve if the physicians find a better combination of medications.

- ☐ Your loved one may need a court order to release them from the psychiatric facility.

- ☐ Your loved one will likely have a harder time finding another long-term care facility to take them after their release from the psychiatric facility.

Many individuals with Alzheimer's disease suffer through a period of aggression. Therefore, you and your family may want to be prepared for this by choosing a psychiatric facility that you would like your loved one transported to in case of emergency. Once you have made this choice, notify your loved one's assisted living or long-term care facility of your decision and ask them to honor your wishes should your loved one need to be placed in a psychiatric facility. Questions to ask when choosing a psychiatric facility are listed below.

Checklist: Questions to ask when choosing a psychiatric facility

- ☐ What is the physician-to-patient ratio? What is the nurse-to-patient ratio?

- ☐ Are physicians available for consultations and appointments over the weekend and on holidays? Or will your loved one be required to wait over the weekend or holiday before being assessed?

- ☐ Do the physicians, nurses, and other employees have experience dealing with behaviors of individuals with advanced Alzheimer's disease?

- [ ] Do the physicians have experience successfully finding medication combinations that can control behavioral changes in your loved one without making them lethargic?

- [ ] Does the facility have a standard protocol for dealing with acts of aggression? If so, what is it? Is it something you are comfortable with?

- [ ] What is the facility's policy on solitary confinement?

- [ ] What is the facility's policy on restraints?

- [ ] Does the facility have a history of reported abuse?

- [ ] Does the facility provide opportunities for mental stimulation and physical activity?

- [ ] Will the facility help your loved one with activities of daily living (e.g., bathing, eating, toileting) if your loved one is unable to do this on their own?

- [ ] Will you be allowed to visit your loved one in the psychiatric facility? If so, what are the visiting hours?

- [ ] What is the overall environment of the psychiatric facility? Does it provide a calm atmosphere? Are residents too isolated?

- [ ] What fees are associated with a voluntary vs. involuntary stay at the psychiatric facility?

- [ ] Will the facility accept your loved one's healthcare or long-term care insurance?

- [ ] How close is the psychiatric

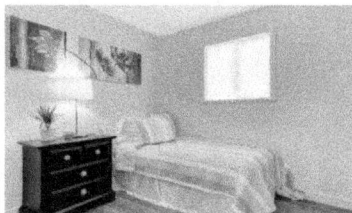

Credit: Iriana Shiyan

facility to your house and your loved one's regular care facility?

☐ What is the facility's policy about releasing your loved one into your care if they were placed in the psychiatric facility by your loved one's assisted living or long-term care facility?

Although having your loved one committed to a psychiatric facility is difficult emotionally, knowing what to expect and being prepared for this possibility will make the transition easier for you. Having a plan in place that your family, your loved one, and your loved one's care facility agree on will make the transition much smoother, and it will prevent any surprises that would cause undue emotional stress.

Chapter 5:
The Moving Process

Moving to a new place can be especially hard on your loved one, no matter what stage of Alzheimer's disease they are in. However, moving is especially hard on individuals in the later stage of Alzheimer's disease. Major moves should be planned long ahead of the move, if possible, in order to ensure the best acclimation to the new environment. When your loved one's surroundings change, this will likely cause a great deal of stress, even if the move goes perfectly. If your loved one does become stressed, their behaviors may become more difficult to manage; alternatively, your loved one could become more withdrawn. Both reactions are entirely normal, as long as they begin to subside in a reasonable amount of time. Keep in mind that acclimating to a new environment does not occur overnight for an individual with Alzheimer's disease. Sometimes it could take your loved one two to three weeks to become comfortable with their new living environment. Depending on how severe your loved one's reaction to the move is, you and other family members may have to avoid visiting for a time to allow your loved one to get used to the new surroundings. This can be difficult for you, and most places will allow you to look in on your loved one so that you know they are safe and well, but without your loved one being able to actually see you. A number of steps can be taken to ensure that the move and subsequent transition are as smooth as possible.

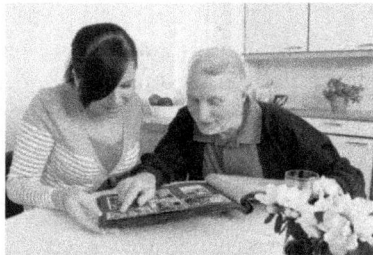

Credit: Lisa S.

Checklist: Easing the transition

- [ ] Bring your loved one to the facility a few times before they move in.

- [ ] Talk to the staff about your loved one's habits, favorite foods, preferred activities, etc.

- [ ] Inform the staff about any daily rituals or schedules your loved one generally follows.

- [ ] Decorate your loved one's room before the move-in day.

- [ ] Bring familiar pictures, blankets, quilts, and decorations for your loved one's new room.

- [ ] If your loved one has a favorite chair or piece of furniture, consider bringing it for their room.

- [ ] Put together scrap books or photo albums with pictures of loved ones, and make sure to label the pictures with names.

- [ ] Decorate the walls with family photos.

- [ ] Move items from your loved one's old home to the new residence when your loved one is not around.

- [ ] Be positive during the move and when talking to your loved one about the new place.

- [ ] Have at least two people at the facility when your loved one moves in; this way, one person can fill out any paperwork and talk to the staff while the other person stays with your loved one.

- [ ] When you leave, try not to make a big production; instead, slip away quietly.

- [ ] Recognize that it will take a few weeks for your loved one to become acclimated to the new surroundings.

☐ If your loved one becomes agitated or stressed when you visit in the first few weeks, consider limiting your visits in order to ease their transition.

Conclusion

Many options exist for living arrangements. Your loved one can usually stay home in the early stages of the disease, but as things progress, they will likely need to move in with a caregiver or move to an assisted living or long-term care facility. These decisions are not easy to make, which is why you should discuss this with your loved one to see what they would prefer while your loved one is still mentally able to make decisions. If you and your family have never had to organize care for a loved one who was ill, the process can be difficult to navigate. Knowing what questions to ask and what features to look for in care facilities can be tremendously valuable. This process is not something you should ever have to go through alone, and there are numerous resources available that can help you organize care for your loved one. Alzheimer's disease does not only affect the individual who has the disease, it impacts the family and friends of that individual as well.

About the Authors

Laura Town

Laura Town has authored numerous publications of special interest to the aging population. She has expertise in the field of finance as a co-author on Finance: Foundations of Financial Institutions and Management published by John Wiley and Sons, and she has contributed to several online nursing courses and texts. She has also written for the American Medical Writers Association, and her work has been published by the American Society of Journalists and Authors. As an editor, Laura has worked with Pearson Education, Prentice Hall, McGraw-Hill Higher Education, John Wiley and Sons, and the University of Pennsylvania to create both on-ground and online courses and texts. She is the past president of the Indiana chapter of the American Medical Writers Association (AMWA).

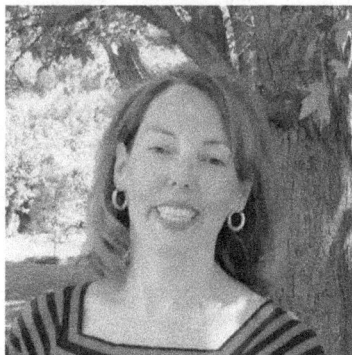

Karen Hoffman

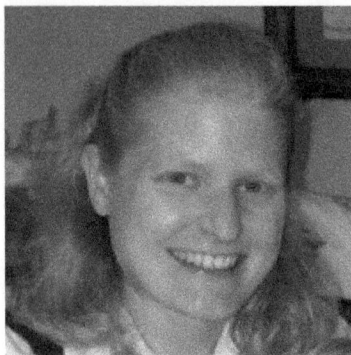

Karen Hoffman received a Ph.D. in Pharmacology from the Department of Pharmacology and Experimental Neurosciences at the University of Nebraska Medical Center in Omaha, NE, where she was the recipient of an American Heart Association fellowship and several regional and national awards for her research on G protein-coupled receptor signaling in airways. She then pursued post-doctoral research projects at the University of North Carolina-Chapel Hill and the University of Kansas Medical Center, again receiving fellowships from the PhRMA Foundation and the American Heart Association, respectively. She has published research in the American Journal of Pathology, Journal of Biological Chemistry, and Journal of Pharmacology and Experimental Therapeutics. In 2012, Karen joined the editorial staff at WilliamsTown Communications, an editing firm that specializes in educational products for undergraduate- and graduate-level students. At WTC, Karen specializes in producing educational products related to the sciences and healthcare. In addition, Karen is board-certified for editing life sciences (BELS-certified).

A Note from the Authors

Thank you for purchasing our book! Worldwide, over 40 million people suffer from Alzheimer's disease, and that number is expected to increase significantly within the next 15 years. In the United States, 5 million people have the disease, and that is expected to triple by the year 2050.

Despite these large numbers, you may feel alone. I (Laura) know that when I started caring for my father, who had early-onset Alzheimer's disease, I felt alone. Although my father has passed away, I am haunted by what he suffered and how difficult it was to care for him. However, now I know that there are people, resources, and organizations that can help others going through this same struggle.

We recognize that caregivers have emotional, physical, and financial challenges. We hope that the information in the *Alzheimer's Roadmap* series will ease some of your stress. The steps included in this book can help you recognize the signs that a new living situation is needed, as well as aid you in assessing that living situation for safety and quality. All of the steps may not apply to every situation, but they will stimulate your thinking and get you progressing forward in the moving process. In addition, we have included resources at the end of each book to provide additional information to help you through this process.

If you have any questions for us, feel free to post them on Laura Town's Amazon Author Central page or reach out to the authors via twitter: @laurawtown. We would appreciate it if you would take the time to review our book on Amazon, as our book's visibility on Amazon depends on reviews.

Additional Titles from Laura Town and Karen Hoffman

Alzheimer's Roadmap series:

Long-Term Care Insurance, Power of Attorney, Wealth Management, and Other First Steps

Dementia, Alzheimer's Disease Stages, Treatment Options, and Other Medical Considerations

Advance Directives, Durable Power of Attorney, Wills, and Other Legal Considerations

Coping with Dementia

Enhancing Activities of Daily Living

Home Safety Checklist Guide and Caregiver Resources for Medication Safety, Driving, and Wandering

Paying for Healthcare and Other Financial Considerations

Home Care, Long-term Care, Memory Care Units, and Other Living Arrangements

Caregiver Resources: From Independence to a Memory Care Unit

Nutrition for Brain Health: Fighting Dementia

Final Steps: End of Life Care for Dementia

Other titles:

How to Save Money on Healthcare

Where Should Mom Live?

Save Money, Live Healthy

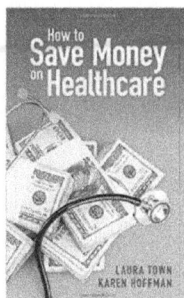

How to Save Money on Healthcare provides answers to the following questions and more:

- **What types of insurance are available to me?** Explore public and private insurance options, learn how they work, and find out who is eligible for them.
- **How can I use my personal savings to pay for care?** Learn about the types of personal wealth, the rules associated with them, and the way they are used to pay for healthcare.
- **What out-of-pocket alternatives exist?** Discover different options to help pay your out-of-pocket medical expenses without draining your savings.
- **How can I manage my medical bills?** Find out how to detect and correct billing errors and what your options are if you are unable to pay your medical bills.

Resources

Alzheimer's Association and Home Services
Phone: 1-800-272-3900
Website: http://www.alz.org/care/

Alzheimer's Association and Caregiver Support Groups
Website: http://www.alz.org/care/alzheimers-dementia-support-groups.asp

Caring Bridge
Website: http://www.caringbridge.org/
This website will help you to coordinate caregiving help with family and friends.

Eldercare Locator
Website: https://eldercare.acl.gov/Public/Index.aspx
This website will help you to find long and short-term care facilities in your area.

National Care Planning Council
Website:
http://www.longtermcarelink.net/a7nursinghome.htm
This website has links to care providers, services, and advisors broken down by state.

Nursing Home Compare
Website:
http://www.medicare.gov/nursinghomecompare/search.html
This website provides information about every nursing home in the country that is Medicare or Medicaid certified.

Senior Living
Website: http://www.seniorliving.org/lifestyles/memory-care/
This website provides a list of long-term, short-term, and

memory care facilities in your area, as well as resources for local homecare services.

Meals on Wheels Association of America
1550 Crystal Drive, Suite 1004
Arlington, VA 22202
Phone: 888-998-6325
Fax: 703-548-5274
Email: info@mealsonwheelsamerica.org
Website: http://www.mealsonwheelsamerica.org/
Website to find a Meals on Wheels in your area:
http://www.mealsonwheelsamerica.org/signup/aboutmea
lsonwheels/find-programs

Caregiver Agreement Examples:

http://co.genesee.ny.us/docs/OfficefortheAging/Caregiv
er_contract_Sample_Agreement_for_Privately_Paid_Ind_.
pdf
http://www.maine.gov/dhhs/ofi/documents/LTC-
Personal-Support-Agreement.pdf
https://www.examples.com/business/personal-care-
agreement.html

Information Resources:

Alzheimer's Association
225 N. Michigan Ave., Fl. 17
Chicago, IL 60601-7633
Phone: 800-272-3900
Fax: 866-699-1246
Email: info@alz.org
Website: http://www.alz.org

Alzheimer's Foundation of America
322 Eighth Ave., 7th fl.
New York, NY 10001
Phone: 866-232-8484
Fax: 646-638-1546
Website: https://alzfdn.org/

Alzheimer's Roadmap series
Purchase on Amazon:
Long-Term Care Insurance, Power of Attorney, Wealth Management, and Other First Steps
Dementia, Alzheimer's Disease Stages, Treatment Options, and Other Medical Considerations
Advance Directives, Durable Power of Attorney, Wills, and Other Legal Considerations
Paying for Healthcare and Other Financial Considerations
Coping with Dementia
Enhancing Activities of Daily Living
Home Safety Checklist Guide and Caregiver Resources for Medication Safety, Driving, and Wandering
Nutrition for Brain Health: Fighting Dementia
Caregiver Resources: From Independence to a Memory Care Unit
Final Steps: End of Life Care for Dementia

Reference List

Administration on Aging. (2017). Home health care. Retrieved from https://acl.gov/sites/default/files/news%202017-03/Home_Health_Care.pdf

Aging Life Care Association. (n.d.). What you need to know. Retrieved from https://www.aginglifecare.org/ALCA/About_Aging_Life_Care/ALCA/About_Aging_Life_Care/What_you_need_to_know.aspx

Alzheimer's Association. (2019). Retrieved from http://www.alz.org/

Alzheimer's Foundation of America. (2017). Excellence in design: Optimal living space for people with Alzheimer's disease and related dementias. Retrieved from https://alzfdn.org/wp-content/uploads/2017/11/Excellence-in-Design-white-paper-June-2014.pdf

A Place for Mom. (2019). Assisted living residence checklist. Retrieved from https://www.aplaceformom.com/planning-and-advice/articles/assisted-living-resident-checklist

Centers for Disease Control and Prevention. (2016, March 11). Nursing home care. Retrieved from https://www.cdc.gov/nchs/fastats/nursing-home-care.htm

Cleveland Clinic. (2019.) Caregiving: Recognizing burnout. Retrieved from https://my.clevelandclinic.org/health/diseases/9225-caregiving-recognizing-burnout

Cleveland Clinic. (2019.) Caregiving: When your stress turns into depression. Retrieved from https://my.clevelandclinic.org/health/diseases/11873-caregiving-when-your-stress-turns-into-depression

Department of Health and Human Services. (2015). Nursing home data compendium 2015 edition. https://www.cms.gov/Medicare/Provider-Enrollment-and-Certification/CertificationandComplianc/Downloads/nursinghomedatacompendium_508-2015.pdf

Family Caregiver Alliance. (2017). Personal care agreements: How to

compensate a family member for providing care. Retrieved from
https://caregiver.org/personal-care-agreements

Fisher Center for Alzheimer's Research Foundation. (2019). Assisted
living facilities. Retrieved from http://www.alzinfo.org/08/treatment-
care/assisted-living-facilities

Gross, J. (2008, October 6). Why hire a Geriatric Care Manager? *The
New York Times*. Retrieved from
http://newoldage.blogs.nytimes.com/2008/10/06/why-hire-a-geriatric-
care-
manager/?_php=true&_type=blogs&_php=true&_type=blogs&_php=
true&_type=blogs&_php=true&_type=blogs&_r=3&

Howley, E. K. (2019, October 11). Nursing home facts and statistics.
U.S. News and World Report. Retrieved from
https://health.usnews.com/health-news/best-nursing-
homes/articles/nursing-home-facts-and-statistics

Mayo Clinic. (2019). Retrieved from http://www.mayoclinic.org/

Meals on Wheels America. (2018.) What we deliver. Retrieved from
https://www.mealsonwheelsamerica.org/learn-more/what-we-deliver

Medicare.gov. (2018). Your guide to choosing a nursing home or other
long-term care. Retrieved from
https://www.medicare.gov/pubs/pdf/02174-Nursing-Home-Other-
Long-Term-Services.pdf

National Institute on Aging. (n.d.). Alzheimer's Caregiving. Retrieved
from https://www.nia.nih.gov/health/alzheimers/caregiving

National Institute on Aging. (n.d.). Everyday care for Alzheimer's.
Retrieved from https://www.nia.nih.gov/health/topics/everyday-care-
alzheimers

Vitus Healthcare. (n.d.). Signs of caregiver burnout and how to prevent
it. Retrieved from https://www.vitas.com/resources/caregiving/signs-
of-caregiver-burnout

SeniorLiving.org. (n.d.). Caregiver burnout 101: Causes, signs,
prevention and solution tips. Retrieved from
https://www.seniorliving.org/caregiving/burnout/

Treatment Advocacy Center. (2018). Know the laws in your state. Retrieved from https://www.treatmentadvocacycenter.org/component/content/article/183-in-a-crisis/1596-know-the-laws-in-your-state

Continue reading to see a selection from another Omega Press title, available now on Amazon.

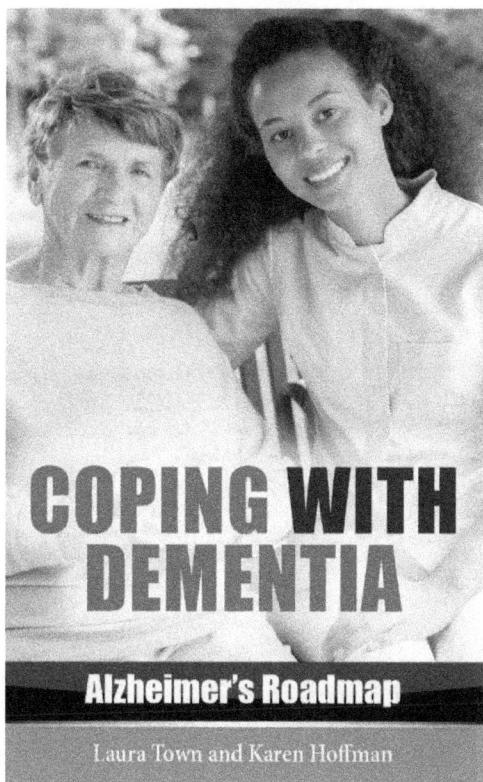

Coping with Dementia

People, whether they be friends or strangers, will be sympathetic when you tell them that a loved one has dementia. Not knowing how to respond, people will try to find something positive to say about your tragedy—and dementia is tragic. The one comment that bothered me (Laura) the most, although the intention behind it was good, was that at least my father "doesn't know what's happening to him." This is completely false. My dad, in the early and even in the mid stages, knew what was happening. Yes, he couldn't articulate it all the time. Yes, he could not go into detail about the functions of the brain or give a scientific explanation of what was happening. But he knew that he could no longer complete simple tasks. He cried when he could no longer drive. He was enraged when he could not remember the names of his relatives. And he sank into a deep depression when he had to start wearing adult diapers. Even in the late stages when dad was living in a locked dementia unit and before he became nonverbal, my father pointed to adults rocking baby dolls and said to me that he wished he wasn't one of "those people."

Dad's doctor told me that if you've seen one case of Alzheimer's disease, it just means that you've seen one case of Alzheimer's disease, meaning that all cases are different. Perhaps some people slide straight from complete cognition to the late stages of Alzheimer's disease and truly do not have any frustration while being in the throes of the disease, but I have never heard of this.

So people with dementia do know, on a

fundamental level, what is happening. That doesn't mean that they know it every day, or even every hour, or become obsessed with their declining health. Dad still had happy moments. He still enjoyed taking walks, listening to music, seeing his grandsons, and eating cupcakes. As long as he was able, I still took him out to restaurants for lunch and dinner or brought him to my house. And although he wasn't particularly religious, he enjoyed visits with the ministers and volunteers who came and read the Bible to him. The challenge is to find what your loved one enjoys and then try to incorporate the enjoyment of it into as many moments of their life as you are able. If you are the one suffering from dementia, then think about what gives you pleasure and find a way to do those things as often as you are able.

When your loved one is diagnosed with Alzheimer's disease or another type of dementia, the emotional effect on the whole family is tremendous. As much as possible, the person with dementia has to come to terms with living with a terminal degenerative disease. They must reckon with a failing memory as well as an increasing reliance on others while also dealing with a society that may feel they have lost their value. Once they enter middle- and later-stage dementia, the disease will begin to affect emotional responses as well as the ability to communicate.

Caregivers, family, and friends of the person with dementia must also process powerful emotions about the news. If your parent, spouse, or other loved one is diagnosed with dementia, you might experience grief over your loved one's loss of memory as well as confusion and stress over practical medical, legal, and financial issues. Your family will likely face some major challenges as you collectively adapt to meet the new needs of the person with dementia. Most significantly, the day-to-day stress of caregiving can take a profound toll on your physical and mental well-being. Being a caregiver affects all parts of your life—personal, professional, and financial—and you may feel that you don't have more than a few minutes to yourself each day. This daily stress can continue for years—sometimes a decade or longer—with serious health implications for you and your family. Studies have found that caregivers' own health problems can be caused or exacerbated by the constant stress of providing care. Studies have also shown that stressed caregivers effectively age faster than people without chronic caregiving responsibilities. According to an American Association of Retired Persons (AARP) report from 2015, 34.2 million Americans provided unpaid care to an adult age 50 or older in the prior 12 months. According to the same report, caregivers spend an average of 24.4 hours a week providing care, with nearly a quarter spending 41 hours or more on care each week, and those caring for a spouse or partner spending 44.6 hours a week. That's an enormous time investment that leaves significantly less time for paid employment and leisure activities. It's easy to see from this how easily caregiving can become all-consuming for the people who provide it.

This book examines the emotional fallout of dementia, and specifically how people with the disease, their caregivers, and their non-caregiver family and friends can cope with that fallout. You'll read about the stages of the disease and how to cope with the common changes at each step. You'll also read about problems that often accompany a terminal chronic illness such as Alzheimer's disease—depression, anxiety, anger, guilt, sleep disturbances, and suicide risk—and how to respond healthily to each of these problems. You'll also get tips and advice for how to support others over the course of dementia: the loved one with the disease, other caregivers, and other family and friends. Although there are different types of dementia including Alzheimer's disease, our checklists should be applicable regardless of the specific diagnosis, and so "dementia" is the term used throughout this book for Alzheimer's disease and other types.

Emotional Considerations for the Individual with Dementia

Dementia destroys the cognitive function of the individual with the disease. Its effects are catastrophic. The reality is that if you have dementia, you will not only lose the ability to think and remember clearly. You will experience extreme behavioral and emotional changes as the disease progresses, will no longer recognize family members or close friends, and may even develop irrational fears and paranoias. Everyone experiences a loss of function and independence as they age. This is often an emotional struggle. But for people with dementia, these normal changes are compounded in every way and are accompanied by other fundamental changes in how they think, speak, and act.

If you have been diagnosed with dementia, all of this will be painful and overwhelming to confront. This is why the first thing you need to do when you are diagnosed, the only thing you need to do, is allow yourself to experience your emotions. This will be different for every person, but this process is very likely to be similar to the stages of grief as defined by the psychiatrist Elisabeth Kübler-Ross: denial, anger, bargaining, depression, and, finally, acceptance. Give yourself the time and permission to experience and move through these emotions. If you need to feel angry, feel angry. If you need to feel depressed, feel depressed. Try not to lash out at others, but experience all the emotions it's natural to feel at this time. Try to talk to other people about how you feel and try not to isolate yourself, but at the same time, do what you need to do. Don't be ashamed of anything you feel right now. Your emotions are telling you what you need. Listen. There will be a time for understanding and for making important decisions, but that time is not when you are first diagnosed. This time is for you to figure out a way to confront this disease that seems most natural to you.

Once you have experienced the emotions you need to experience, then it is time to seek help to get some of the legal and financial documents you need in place. You won't want to think about this, but it is important to do now while you can still think clearly and make these important decisions for yourself. You can get help with this from your loved ones and learn the basics steps by reading *Long-Term Care Insurance, Power of Attorney, Wealth Management, and Other First Steps*. These first steps come with their own emotional struggles, and it's okay to embrace and experience those emotions, too. You're not alone in this, and whenever you need it, ask for help along the way.

The next two sections examine how to begin understanding the progression of dementia and coping with the diagnosis from the perspective of the individual with the disease. Then the following section turns to the caregiver to suggest ways that caregivers can help with that coping.

How Dementia Progresses

One thing that may help you if you have been diagnosed with dementia is to learn what the disease is and what it does. Probably the best way to approach understanding dementia is to learn what you should expect as the disease progresses. Although the effects of dementia and how it progresses are different for everyone who has it, generally people with dementia experience a gradual worsening of symptoms over time. In the early stages, memory loss and reduction of ability to function are minor and very gradual, but in the later phases, people with dementia lose the ability to participate in give-and-take conversation and react to stimuli. If you have dementia, activities you used to do easily, such as balancing a checkbook or keeping track of your keys, will become gradually more difficult. The checklist below focuses on the early changes to expect.

Checklist: Early changes to expect with dementia

☐ Disruptive memory loss, such as forgetting information you learned recently and important dates and events. You may ask for the same information again and again, but you may not remember that you've already asked for it.

☐ Difficulty solving problems, such planning an event and keeping track of bills. Working with numbers or following processes with many steps may become especially difficult.

☐ Being confused about time and place. You may have trouble remembering what day it is, why you are where you are and what you were doing, or what is happening right now.

☐ Misplacing things, such as not finding car keys where you expect them to be.

☐ Difficulty performing familiar work or personal tasks. This may make it challenging or impossible to continue working if you are not retired.

☐ Problems with self-expression, such as difficulty organizing thoughts or finding the right words to say what you mean. This may make it difficult for you to follow conversations or to take an active part in them.

☐ Impaired judgment that compromises decision making. This may be difficult for you to be aware of, but if you think you've paid for a good or service you haven't received, you notice charges that don't look right to you in your credit card statements, or you receive strange bills, ask for help from your caregivers in understanding what concerns you.

☐ Changes in mood and personality, such as depression, anxiety, or sudden and unpredictable irritability and anger. You may become socially withdrawn, even if you are normally very social, and you may lose motivation to complete tasks, especially challenging ones.

How to Cope if You Have Been Diagnosed with Dementia

If you feel embarrassed by your symptoms and are afraid to talk to others or ask for help, you are not alone. Many people with dementia experience this. However, trying to cover up the symptoms can be very stressful, and eventually it's impossible to cover up the signs. Instead, you should try to integrate changes from the disease into daily life while remaining as active and engaged as possible. If you have been diagnosed, remember to be flexible, fine-tune your approach from day to day, and ask for help. Although some people stigmatize the need to depend on others as weak and parasitic, it is wrong to view relationships this way, especially your relationships with close family and friends. People help one another not just out of a sense of obligation but also to find meaning and purpose in their own lives. If you let other people help you, you can better cope with the disease, and you may also help them cope better with it as well by giving them a way to deal with it. Remember: You and the ones who love and care for you are all in this together.

Checklist: How to cope with a diagnosis of dementia

- ☐ Research dementia and discuss your feelings and findings with loved ones.

- ☐ Involve family and friends in your efforts to learn all you can about dementia.

- ☐ Ask all medical providers to explain medical terms and instructions that you find confusing or do not remember. Encourage a close family member or friend to assist you in these efforts, helping you take note of anything important for you to know about your diagnosis.

☐ Find out what support services are available in your community. Local organizations may offer everything from transportation help to peer counseling.

☐ Decide who your primary caregivers should be and, with their help, begin creating and organizing a daily routine for yourself.

☐ If you feel overwhelmed with depression, anxiety, and stress following your diagnosis, don't hesitate to seek out a mental health provider. Meeting with a mental health professional early in the course of the disease can help you cope better as the condition worsens. For information on finding a mental health provider, see the Resources at the end of this book.

www.ingramcontent.com/pod-product-compliance
Lightning Source LLC
Chambersburg PA
CBHW021132020426
42331CB00005B/742